TOP 20

BODY WEIGHT EXERCISES

10 Minute intense fully body workouts to lose weight, build muscle with no equipment.

TABLE OF CONTENTS

CHAPTER 1

INTRODUCTION

As a full-time athletic trainer, I understand the challenges of finding time for exercise amidst a busy schedule. The demands of daily life, the hustle and bustle, and the expenses associated with gym memberships or specialized equipment often leave us feeling overwhelmed and deterred from working out. I wanted to write a book that addresses these obstacles and provides a solution that fits seamlessly into any lifestyle.

This book is designed to show you that no matter how hectic your schedule, you can carve out just 10 minutes a day for movement. Bodyweight exercises are efficient and can be done anywhere—at home, in the office, or outdoors—without needing equipment. I aim to simplify fitness and make it accessible to everyone, regardless of time constraints or financial limitations.

I am excited to present this easy-to-follow guide that demystifies bodyweight training and offers practical, efficient workouts. This book lets you stay active, build strength, and improve your overall health without the stress of fitting a gym session into your already packed day.

I recommend that you consult with your physician before starting any workout program to ensure that it is suitable for you.

CHAPTER 2

WHY BODYWEIGHT EXERCISES AND WORKOUTS

The Power of Simplicity

Bodyweight training is an effective and efficient way to build strength, improve cardiovascular health, and enhance flexibility without expensive equipment or a gym membership. These exercises can be performed anywhere, making them ideal for those with busy lifestyles or limited access to fitness facilities.

Benefits of Bodyweight Training

- **Accessibility**: Suitable for all fitness levels, from beginners to advanced athletes.
- **Cost-Effective**: No need for costly gym memberships or equipment.
- **Versatility**: This can be performed anywhere, anytime.

- **Comprehensive Fitness**: Engages multiple muscle groups, improves balance coordination, and promotes cardiovascular health.
- **Sustainability**: Encourages lifelong fitness habits.

Different Types of Training

Understanding the various training methods can help you maximize your results and keep your routines fresh and exciting when it comes to bodyweight workouts. Here, we'll explore different types of training and how they can be applied to bodyweight exercises.

Circuit Training

Circuit training is an efficient and comprehensive workout method that combines strength training and cardiovascular exercise. In a circuit, you perform a series of exercises in a specific sequence with minimal rest between each exercise. Typically, a circuit includes five to ten exercises, each performed for a set amount of time or a particular number of repetitions. After completing all the circuit exercises, you rest briefly before repeating the entire sequence. This method not only improves cardiovascular fitness but also enhances muscular endurance. Imagine a circuit with push-ups, squats, planks, jumping jacks, and lunges. Moving quickly from one exercise to the next keeps your heart rate elevated and engages multiple muscle groups.

Eccentric Training

Eccentric training focuses on the lengthening phase of a muscle contraction. This type of training emphasizes the slow and controlled lowering portion of an exercise, which increases muscle strength and hypertrophy. For instance, when performing a push-up, you would reduce your body slowly, taking three to five seconds to descend, before pushing back up more quickly. Eccentric training can be efficient in bodyweight exercises like squats, push-ups, and pull-ups. Incorporating eccentric movements enhances muscle control, stability, and overall strength.

Isometric Training

Isometric training involves holding a muscle contraction in a static position without changing the muscle's length or the joint's angle. This method is excellent for building muscular endurance and stability. During an isometric exercise, you hold the position where the muscle is under tension for a specific period, typically between 20 to 60 seconds. Joint isometric exercises include planks, wall sits, and holding the bottom position of a push-up. This type of training can improve joint stability and is particularly useful for rehabilitation and injury prevention.

High-Intensity Interval Training (HIIT)

High-Intensity Interval Training, or HIIT, is a popular training method that alternates between short bursts of intense exercise and periods of rest or low-intensity exercise. HIIT is highly effective for maximizing calorie burn in a short amount of time. During a HIIT session, you might perform an exercise at maximum effort for 20 to 40 seconds, followed by a rest period or lower-intensity activity for 10 to 20 seconds. This cycle is repeated for a set duration or number of rounds. HIIT workouts, such as 30 seconds of burpees followed by 15 seconds of rest, are known for improving cardiovascular fitness, metabolic rate, and muscle strength.

Plyometric Training

Plyometric training involves explosive movements that increase power and strength by utilizing the muscles' stretch-shortening cycle. These exercises require rapid stretching followed by explosive contractions, making them ideal for developing muscle power and speed. Plyometric exercises include jump squats, box jumps, and burpees. Incorporating plyometrics into your bodyweight routines can enhance athletic performance by improving coordination, agility, and cardiovascular fitness.

Functional Training

Functional training focuses on exercises that improve everyday movements and activities by engaging multiple muscle groups and emphasizing natural movement patterns. This type of training prepares your body for daily tasks or specific sports activities. Functional exercises often involve compound movements that engage the core and improve overall stability and strength. Examples of functional training exercises include lunges with a twist, multi-directional lunges, and exercises that mimic daily activities. Improving functional strength enhances your ability to perform everyday tasks and reduces the risk of injuries.

Tabata Training

Tabata training is a specific form of HIIT that consists of 20 seconds of ultra-intense exercise followed by 10 seconds of rest, repeated for four minutes (eight rounds). This training method is highly effective for increasing aerobic and anaerobic capacity. During a Tabata session, you perform an exercise at maximum intensity for 20 seconds, rest for 10 seconds, and repeat the cycle.

Tabata workouts, such as 20 seconds of mountain climbers followed by 10 seconds of rest, are designed to maximize calorie burn and improve conditioning quickly.

Superset Training

Superset training involves performing two back-to-back exercises with no rest in between, typically targeting opposing or the same muscle group. This method increases workout intensity and volume, making it an efficient way to build muscle and strength. In a superset, you might perform push-ups followed immediately by inverted rows. Superset training saves time and can enhance muscle endurance and strength by keeping your muscles under constant tension.

You can create a diverse and effective fitness program by incorporating these various training methods into your bodyweight workouts. Each technique offers unique benefits, whether you want to build strength, improve cardiovascular health, increase flexibility, or enhance overall fitness. Understanding and applying these training techniques will help you achieve your fitness goals and keep your workouts engaging and challenging.

CHAPTER 3

UPPER BODY EXERCISES

Essential Upper Body Moves

Push-Ups: Targets chest, shoulders, and triceps.

Start in a plank position with your hands slightly wider than shoulder-width apart and directly under your shoulders. Your body should form a straight line from head to heels, with feet together or slightly apart. Tighten your core to maintain this alignment throughout the exercise.

Lowering Phase: Inhale as you bend your elbows, lowering your chest toward the floor. Keep your elbows at a 45-degree angle to your body and lower yourself until your chest is just above the ground.

Pushing Phase: Exhale as you press through your hands to extend your elbows and push your body back up to the starting position. Keep your core engaged and maintain a straight body alignment, avoiding locking your elbows at the top.

Common Mistakes to Avoid:

- **Sagging hips**: Keep your core tight to prevent this.
- **Flaring elbows**: Maintain a 45-degree angle to protect your shoulders.
- **Incomplete range of motion**: Lower your chest until it's just above the floor.

Tips for Beginners:

- **Knee Push-Ups**: Perform the exercise with knees on the floor.

- **Incline Push-Ups**: Use a raised surface like a bench or table to reduce resistance.

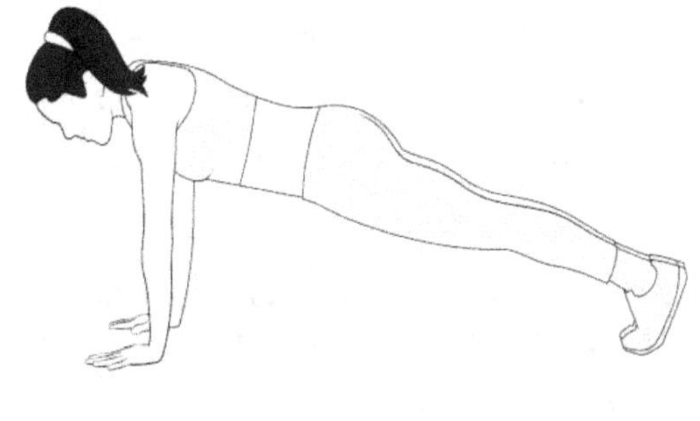

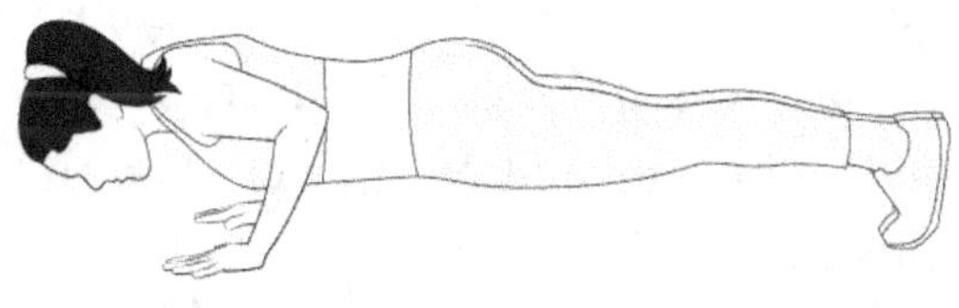

Dips: Focuses on triceps and shoulders.

Starting Position:

Begin by sitting on the edge of a sturdy bench or chair with your hands gripping the edge, fingers pointing forward. Slide your hips off the bench, supporting your weight with your arms. Extend your legs straight out in front of you, keeping your feet together and heels on the ground. Your body should be close to the bench, with your arms straight and shoulders relaxed.

Execution:

Lowering Phase: Inhale as you slowly bend your elbows, lowering your body toward the ground. Your elbows should bend to about a 90-degree angle, keeping them close to your body to emphasize the triceps. Lower yourself until your upper arms are parallel to the floor.

Pushing Phase: Exhale as you press through your hands to extend your elbows, pushing your body back up to the starting position. Keep your core engaged and your back close to the bench throughout the movement.

Common Mistakes to Avoid:

- **Flaring elbows**: Keep your elbows close to your body to focus on the triceps and avoid shoulder strain.
- **Inadequate range of motion**: Lower yourself until your upper arms parallel the ground.
- **Hips too far from the bench**: Keep your back close to the bench to maintain proper form and reduce stress on the shoulders.

Tips for Beginners:

- **Bent-Knee Dips**: If straight-leg dips are too challenging, bend your knees and keep your feet flat on the floor to reduce the amount of body weight you're lifting.
- **Reduced Range of Motion**: Initially, lower yourself only partway down, gradually increasing the depth as you build strength.

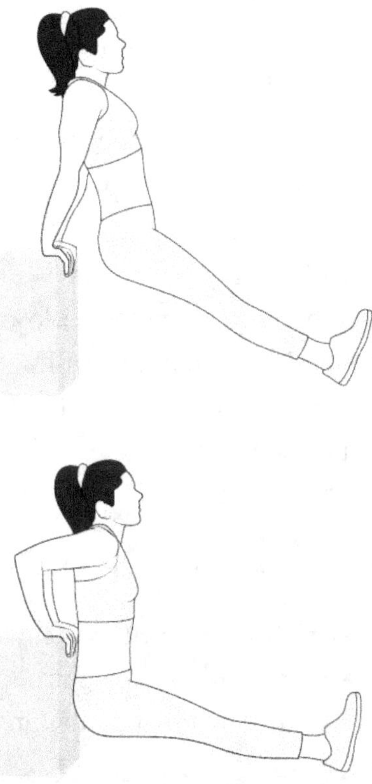

Pull-Ups: Engages back, shoulders, and biceps.

Starting Position:

Find a sturdy pull-up bar. Grip the bar with your palms facing away from you (overhand grip) and your hands shoulder-width apart. Hang from the bar with your arms extended and your feet off the ground. Engage your core to stabilize your body and keep your shoulders down and back.

Execution:

Pulling Up (Concentric Movement):

- **Inhale and Prepare:** Engage your core and back muscles as you prepare to pull yourself up.
- **Pull Up:** Exhale as you pull your body upward, leading with your chest. Focus on driving your elbows down and back, keeping them close to your body.
- **Chin Over Bar:** Continue pulling until your chin is above the bar. Your chest should be close to the bar, and your shoulder blades should be retracted (squeezed together).

Lowering Phase (Eccentric Movement):

- **Inhale as You Lower:** Slowly lower your body back to the starting position in a controlled manner. Extend your arms fully while maintaining tension in your muscles.
- **Controlled Descent:** Keep your core engaged and avoid swinging or using momentum. Ensure a smooth and steady descent to maximize muscle engagement.

Common Mistakes to Avoid:

- **Using momentum:** Avoid swinging your body or kicking your legs to generate momentum. Focus on using your upper body muscles to perform the movement.
- **Partial range of motion:** Complete each rep by lowering yourself fully and pulling up until your chin is above the bar.

- **Flared elbows:** Keep your elbows close to your body to protect your shoulders and engage the correct muscles.

Tips for Beginners:

- **Assisted Pull-Ups:** Use resistance bands or an assisted pull-up machine to reduce the amount of body weight you need to lift.
- **Negative Pull-Ups:** Focus on the lowering phase by jumping or stepping up to the bar and then slowly lowering yourself down.
- **Chin-Ups:** If they feel easier, start with chin-ups (palms facing towards you), as this grip engages the biceps more.

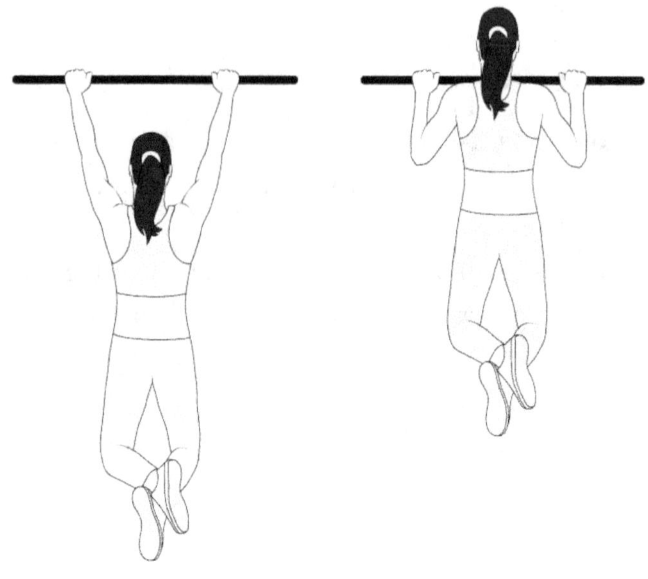

Inchworms: Strengthens shoulders and core.

Starting Position:

Begin by standing with your feet hip-width apart and your arms at your sides. Ensure you have enough space in front of you to walk your hands out.

Execution:

Lowering Phase:

- Inhale as you hinge at your hips, bending forward to place your hands on the floor. If necessary, bend your knees slightly to reach the ground.
- Keeping your core engaged, walk your hands forward, one step at a time until you are in a plank position with your hands directly under your shoulders.

Plank Position:

- Ensure your body forms a straight line from your head to your heels. Your core should be tight, and your shoulders should be over your wrists.
- Hold this position briefly, engaging your shoulders and core.

Returning Phase:

- Exhale as you walk your hands back toward your feet, maintaining a strong core.
- Keep your legs as straight as possible to stretch your hamstrings.
- Once your hands reach your feet, stand up straight to return to the starting position.

Common Mistakes to Avoid:

- **Sagging hips**: Keep your core tight to prevent your hips from dropping while in the plank position.
- **Rounded back**: Maintain a straight back as you bend forward and walk your hands out.

- **Rushing the movement**: Perform the exercise in a controlled manner to maximize muscle engagement.

Tips for Beginners:

- **Bend your knees**: If you have tight hamstrings, bend your knees slightly to reach the floor without straining your lower back.
- **Shorter range of motion**: If a full plank is too challenging, walk your hands out only part way until you build strength and flexibility.

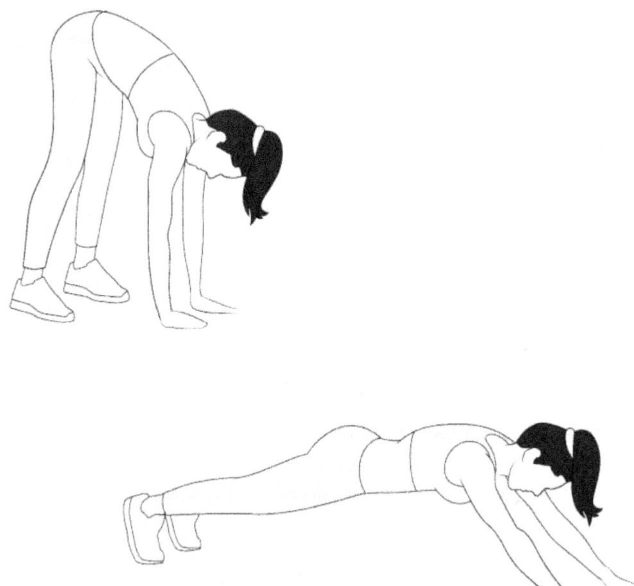

**Pike Push-Ups:** Targets shoulders and upper chest.

Starting Position:

Begin in a downward-facing dog position with your hands shoulder-width apart on the floor and your feet hip-width apart. Your body should form an inverted V shape, with your hips raised toward the ceiling. Keep your arms and legs straight, and ensure your head is between your arms.

Execution:

Lowering Phase:

- Inhale as you bend your elbows and lower your head toward the floor. Keep your elbows pointing outward and maintain the inverted V shape of your body.
- Lower yourself until the top of your head is just above the floor, ensuring that your elbows are bent at about a 90-degree angle.

Pushing Phase:

- Exhale as you push through your hands to straighten your arms and raise your head back to the starting position.
- Focus on engaging your shoulders and triceps as you press up, keeping your core tight to maintain stability.

Common Mistakes to Avoid:

- **Sagging hips**: Keep your hips raised and your core engaged to maintain the inverted V shape.
- **Flaring elbows**: Ensure your elbows are pointing out to the sides, not back, to target the shoulders effectively.

- **Incomplete range of motion**: Lower yourself until your head is just above the floor to maximize the benefits of the exercise.

Tips for Beginners:

- **Elevate your hands**: If a standard pike push-up is too challenging, start with your hands on an elevated surface, like a bench or step, to reduce the intensity.
- **Bend your knees**: If you have tight hamstrings, bend your knees slightly to maintain the proper inverted V shape without straining your lower back.

Advanced Variations

- Diamond Push-Ups
- Clap Push-Ups
- Archer Push-Ups
- Handstand Push-Ups

LOWER BODY EXERCISES

Foundational Lower Body Exercises

**Squats:** Targets quadriceps, hamstrings, and glutes.

Starting Position:

Stand with your feet shoulder-width apart and your toes pointing slightly outward.

Keep your chest up shoulders back, and engage your core to maintain a straight back.

Execution:

Lowering Phase (Eccentric Movement):

- Inhale as you begin to lower your body by bending your hips and knees. Imagine sitting back in a chair.

- Keep your chest up and your back straight as you descend. Your knees should track over your toes without extending past them.
- Lower yourself until your thighs are parallel to the floor or as low as you can go while maintaining good form. Your knees and toes should be in line, and your weight should be distributed evenly across your feet, with a slight emphasis on your heels.

Pushing Phase (Concentric Movement):

- Exhale as you push through your heels to straighten your legs and return to the starting position.
- Keep your chest up and your core engaged as you rise. Ensure that your knees do not cave inward during the ascent.
- Fully extend your hips and knees at the top of the movement, but avoid locking your knees.

Common Mistakes to Avoid:

- **Knees caving inward**: Ensure your knees track over your toes to prevent injury and maximize muscle engagement.
- **Leaning forward**: Keep your chest up and back straight to avoid placing undue stress on your lower back.
- **Heels lifting off the ground**: Distribute your weight evenly across your feet, with an emphasis on pressing through your heels.

Tips for Beginners:

- **Use a chair**: Practice by squatting down to a chair to help with balance and proper depth.
- **Wall squats**: Perform squats with your back against a wall to help maintain proper alignment and support.
- **Partial squats**: Start with partial squats, only lowering halfway, and gradually increase the depth as you build strength and flexibility.

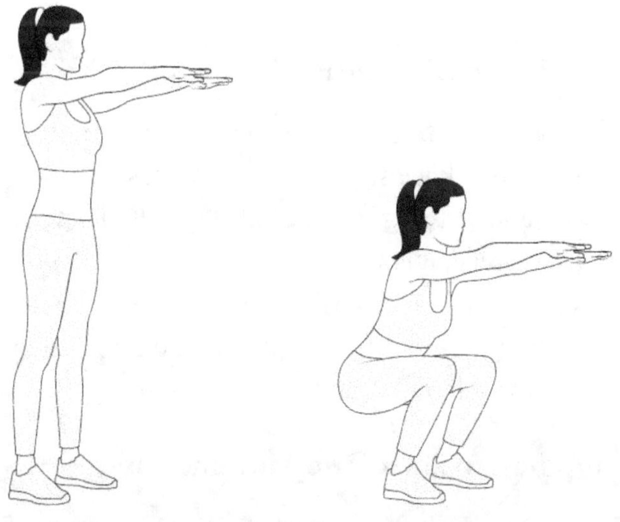

Lunges: Engages quadriceps, glutes, and calves.

Starting Position:

Stand upright with your feet hip-width apart and your hands on your hips or by your sides. Engage your core and keep your chest lifted and shoulders back.

Execution:

Stepping Forward (Initial Movement):

- Take a step forward with your right foot, landing softly on your heel first. The step should be large enough so that when you lower your body, your front knee stays directly above your ankle and does not extend past your toes.

Lowering Phase (Eccentric Movement):

- Inhale as you lower your body by bending both knees. Your back knee should lower towards the floor, stopping just above the ground. Both legs should form roughly 90-degree angles.
- Keep your torso upright and your core engaged. Your front thigh should be parallel to the floor, and your back knee should point directly downward.

Pushing Phase (Concentric Movement):

- Exhale as you push through the heel of your front foot to extend your knees and return to the starting position. Ensure your front knee tracks over your toes and does not cave inward.
- Step back to the starting position, maintaining balance and control.

Alternate Legs:

- Repeat the movement by stepping forward with your left foot and following the same steps.

Common Mistakes to Avoid:

- **Knees caving inward**: Keep your front knee aligned with your toes to avoid injury and maximize muscle engagement.
- **Leaning forward**: Maintain an upright torso throughout the movement to avoid placing stress on your lower back.
- **Short steps**: Ensure your step is large enough to allow your knees to form 90-degree angles without your front knee extending past your toes.

Tips for Beginners:

- **Stationary lunges**: Perform lunges without stepping forward by simply lowering and raising your body while keeping your feet in place.
- **Assisted lunges**: Use a wall or chair for support to help with balance and stability.
- **Partial lunges**: Start with partial lunges, only lowering halfway, and gradually increasing the depth as you build strength and confidence.

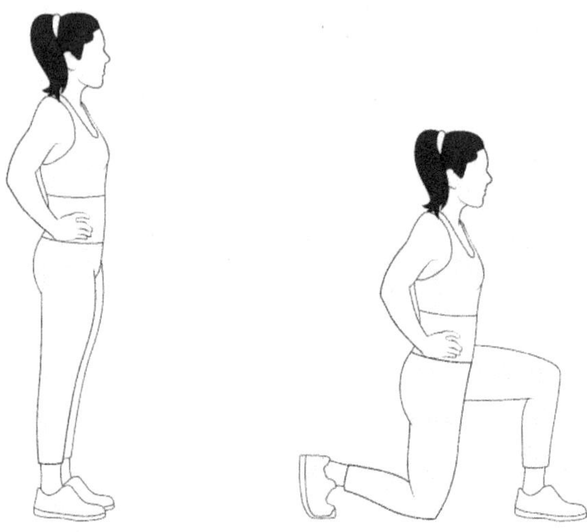

Step-Ups: Strengthens legs and improves balance.

Starting Position:

Stand upright, facing a sturdy bench, step, or box. Ensure the surface is stable and at a height that allows your knee to form a 90-degree angle when your foot is on the step. Place your feet hip-width apart and your hands on your hips or by your sides. Engage your core and keep your chest lifted and shoulders back.

Execution:

Stepping Up (Initial Movement):

- Place your right foot firmly on the bench or step. Ensure your entire foot is on the surface to maintain balance and stability.
- Engage your core and glutes as you press through your right heel to lift your body onto the step. Straighten your right leg, bringing your left foot up to meet your right foot on the bench.

Stepping Down:

- Inhale as you step down with your left foot, lowering it back to the ground. Follow with your right foot, returning to the starting position.
- Maintain control and balance throughout the movement, ensuring a smooth descent.

Alternate Legs:

- Repeat the movement by stepping up with your left foot and following the same steps.

Common Mistakes to Avoid:

- **Incomplete foot placement**: Ensure your entire foot is on the step to avoid slipping and maintain stability.
- **Pushing off with the back foot**: Use your lead leg to lift your body rather than pushing off with the foot on the ground.
- **Leaning forward**: Keep your torso upright to avoid placing undue stress on your lower back.

- **Rushing the movement**: Perform the exercise in a controlled manner to maximize muscle engagement and prevent injury.

Tips for Beginners:

- **Lower step**: Start with a lower step or bench to build strength and confidence before progressing to higher surfaces.

- **Assisted step-ups**: Use a wall or chair for support to help with balance and stability.

- **Partial step-ups**: Begin with partial step-ups, only stepping halfway up, and gradually increase the height as you build strength.

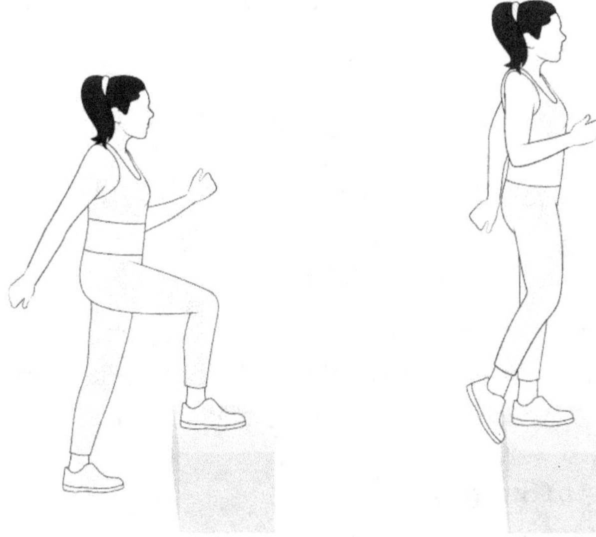

Wall Sits: Builds endurance in the lower body.

Starting Position:

Find a smooth, sturdy wall and stand with your back against it. Your feet should be shoulder-width apart and about 2 feet away from the wall. Ensure your body is aligned, with your back flat against the wall and your shoulders relaxed.

Execution:

Lowering Phase (Eccentric Movement):

- Slowly slide your back down the wall while bending your knees. Continue to slide down until your thighs are parallel to the floor, forming a 90-degree angle at your knees. Your knees should be directly above your ankles, not extending past your toes.

- Keep your feet flat on the ground and distribute your weight evenly across your feet.

Holding Position (Isometric Phase):

- Hold this position while keeping your back flat against the wall and your core engaged. Your hands can rest on your thighs or hang by your sides.

- Maintain this position for the desired amount of time, typically starting with 20-30 seconds and gradually increasing as you build strength and endurance.

Returning to Start:

- Once you have held the position for the desired time, slowly slide your back up the wall to return to the starting position. Straighten your legs and stand up tall.

Common Mistakes to Avoid:

- **Knees extending past toes**: Ensure your knees are directly above your ankles to avoid placing excessive stress on your knees.

- **Leaning forward**: Keep your back flat against the wall to maintain proper alignment and engage your core.

- **Short duration**: Hold the position for the recommended time to maximize muscle engagement and endurance.

Tips for Beginners:

- **Shorter duration**: Start by holding the wall sit for a shorter duration, such as 10-15 seconds, and gradually increase the time as you build strength.

- **Higher position**: If a 90-degree angle is too challenging, begin with a higher position where your thighs are not completely parallel to the floor, and lower yourself as you gain strength and confidence.

- **Supportive surface**: Ensure the wall is smooth and sturdy to provide adequate support during the exercise.

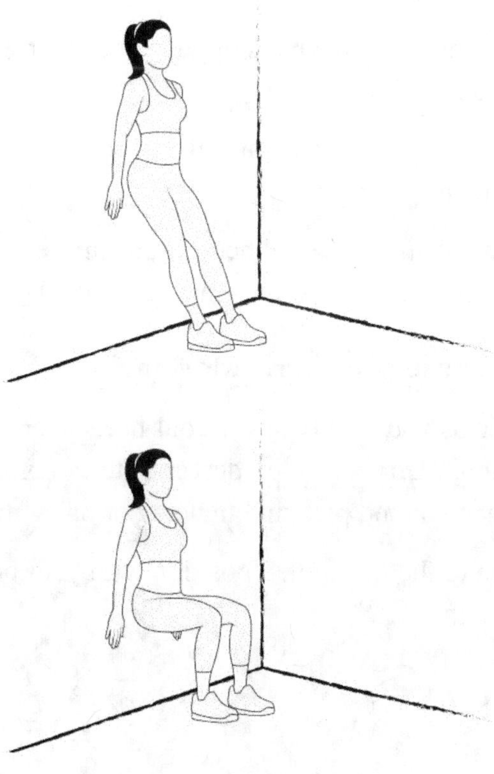

Calf Raises: Focuses on calf muscles.

Starting Position:

Stand upright with your feet hip-width apart. Ensure your body weight is evenly distributed across both feet. You can perform this exercise with your hands resting on your hips, by your sides, or lightly holding onto a wall or chair for balance.

Execution:

Lifting Phase (Concentric Movement):

- Inhale as you prepare to lift. Engage your core to maintain stability and keep your torso upright.

- Slowly rise onto the balls of your feet, lifting your heels as high as possible.

- Focus on squeezing your calf muscles at the top of the movement.

- Ensure your ankles, knees, and hips remain aligned throughout the lift. Avoid leaning forward or backward.

Lowering Phase (Eccentric Movement):

- Exhale as you slowly lower your heels back to the starting position. Control the descent to maximize muscle engagement and prevent bouncing or using momentum.

- Return to the flat-footed position with your heels touching the ground.

Repetition:

- Repeat the movement for the desired number of repetitions. Aim for 10-15 repetitions to start, gradually increasing as you build strength and endurance.

Common Mistakes to Avoid:

- **Bouncing**: Avoid bouncing at the bottom of the movement. Focus on controlled, deliberate movements to engage the calf muscles effectively.

- **Leaning forward or backward**: Keep your torso upright and your body aligned to maintain proper form and prevent strain on other muscles.

- **Inadequate range of motion**: Lift your heels as high as possible and lower them fully to maximize the exercise's effectiveness.

Tips for Beginners:

- **Support for balance**: If you find it challenging to maintain balance, perform calf raises while holding onto a wall or chair for support.

- **Single-leg variation**: Once you're comfortable with the basic calf raise, you can progress to single-leg calf raises to increase the intensity and challenge your balance further.

- **Add resistance**: To further challenge your calf muscles, you can hold dumbbells in your hands or wear a weighted vest.

- **Advanced Movements**
- Pistol Squats
- Jump Squats

- Bulgarian Split Squats

- Single-Leg Deadlifts

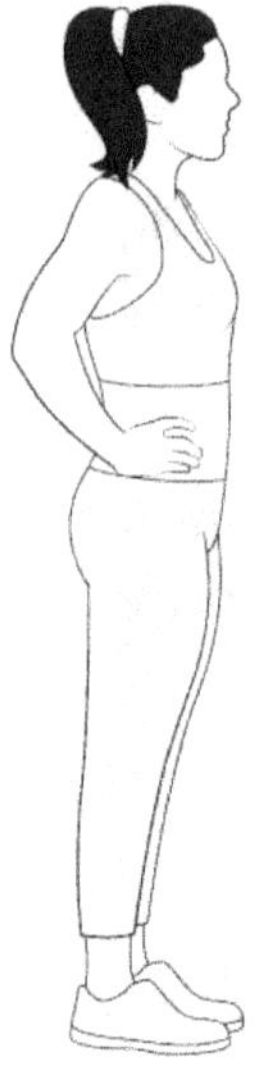
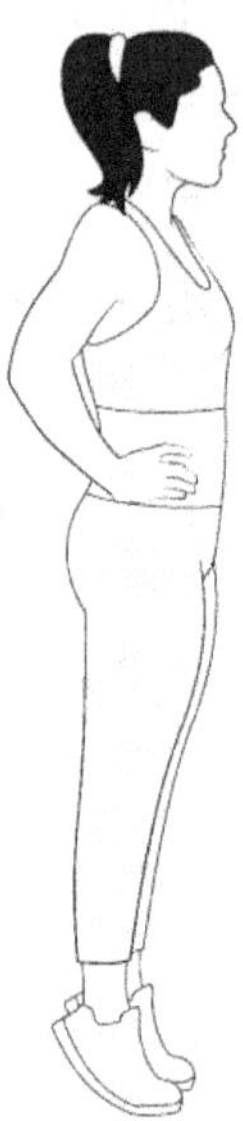

CHAPTER 5

CORE/ABS

Core Essentials

Planks: Engages the entire core.

Starting Position:

Begin by lying face down on the floor. Position your elbows directly under your shoulders and place your forearms on the ground, parallel to each other. Your feet should be hip-width apart with your toes on the ground. Engage your core and lift your body off the ground, creating a straight line from your head to your heels.

Execution:

Holding the Position (Isometric Movement):

- Keep your body straight and rigid, avoiding any sagging or arching of your back. Your head should be in a neutral position, aligned with your spine, and your gaze directed slightly ahead.

- Engage your core by pulling your belly button towards your spine. Squeeze your glutes and tighten your leg muscles to maintain stability.

- Hold this position for the desired amount of time, starting with 20-30 seconds and gradually increasing as you build strength and endurance.

Maintaining Form:

- Ensure your shoulders are directly over your elbows and your forearms are parallel. Keep your shoulders away from your ears, maintaining a relaxed yet firm posture.

- Focus on keeping your hips level and your body in a straight line from head to heels. Avoid letting your hips drop or rise too high.

Common Mistakes to Avoid:

- **Sagging hips**: Keep your core engaged to prevent your hips from dropping, which can strain your lower back.

- **Raised hips**: Avoid lifting your hips too high, which reduces the effectiveness of the exercise.

- **Looking up or down**: Maintain a neutral head position to keep your spine aligned.

Tips for Beginners:

- **Modified plank**: If a full plank is too challenging, start with a modified plank by keeping your knees on the ground while maintaining a straight line from your head to your knees.

- **Shorter duration**: Begin by holding the plank for shorter periods, such as 10-15 seconds, and gradually increase the time as you build strength.

- **Rest breaks**: If you find it difficult to hold the plank continuously, take brief rest breaks and then resume the position to complete the set duration.

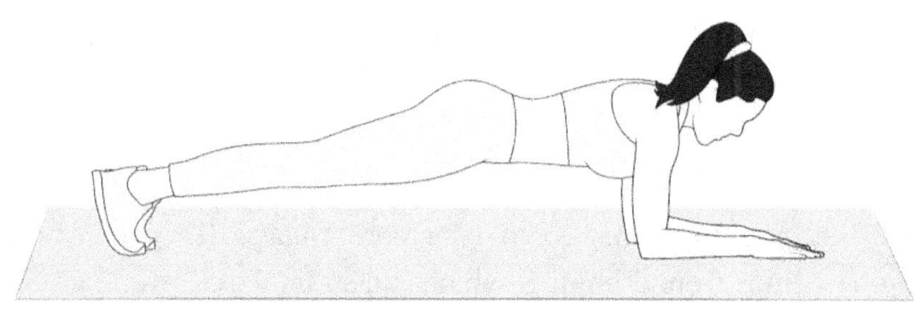

Russian Twists: Targets obliques.

Starting Position:

Sit on the floor with your knees bent and your feet flat on the ground. Lean back slightly to create a 45-degree angle with your torso, ensuring your back is straight and not rounded. Engage your core to maintain this position. Clasp your hands together in front of your chest or hold a weight or medicine ball for added resistance.

Execution:

Twisting Movement:

- Exhale as you twist your torso to the right, bringing your clasped hands or the weight beside your right hip. Your shoulders and arms should move together as a unit, driven by the rotation of your torso.

- Inhale as you return to the center position, keeping your core engaged.

- Exhale again as you twist to the left, bringing your hands or the weight beside your left hip.

Maintaining Form:

- Keep your feet either flat on the ground or, for an added challenge, lift them slightly off the floor while maintaining balance.

- Ensure your movements are controlled and deliberate, avoiding jerky or rushed motions.

- Maintain the 45-degree angle with your torso throughout the exercise to keep constant tension on your core muscles.

Common Mistakes to Avoid:

- **Leaning too far back or forward**: Maintain the 45-degree angle to avoid straining your lower back.

- **Using only your arms**: Ensure the twist comes from your torso and not just your arms moving side to side.

  Inadequate core engagement: Keep your core tight and engaged to maximize the effectiveness of the exercise.

Tips for Beginners:

- **No weight**: Start by performing the Russian twist without any added weight, focusing on perfecting your form.

- **Feet on the ground**: Keep your feet flat on the ground to help maintain balance and stability.

- **Shorter duration**: Perform the exercise for shorter periods or fewer repetitions, gradually increasing as you build strength and endurance.

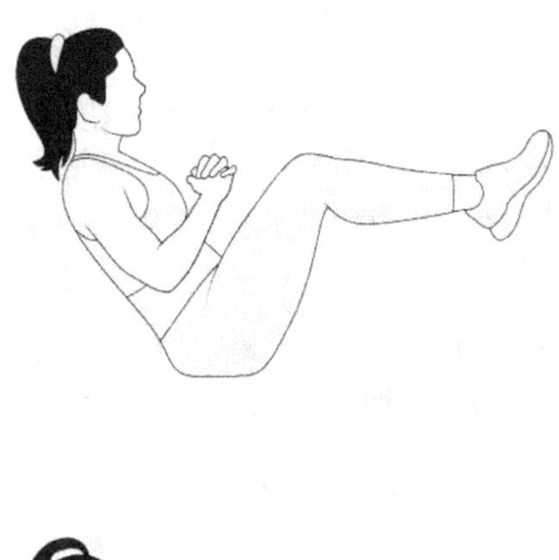

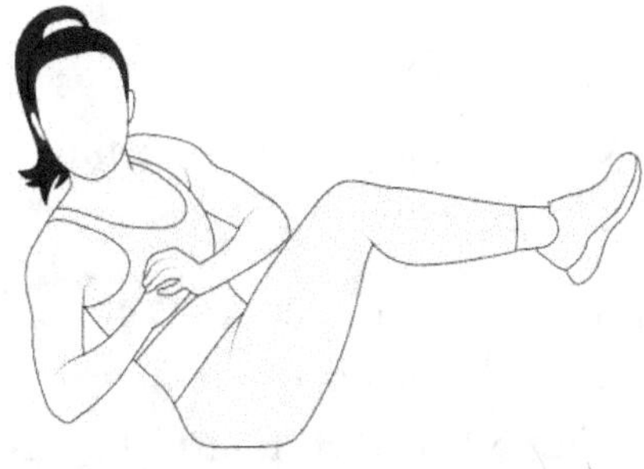

Leg Raises: Strengthens lower abs.

Starting Position:

Lie flat on your back on an exercise mat with your legs extended straight and your arms by your sides, palms facing down. Engage your core by pulling your belly button towards your spine and keep your lower back pressed into the mat.

Execution:

Lifting Phase (Concentric Movement):

- Inhale deeply as you prepare to lift your legs. Keeping your legs straight and together, slowly raise them towards the ceiling. Focus on using your lower abdominal muscles to lift your legs.

- Continue to lift your legs until they form a 90-degree angle with your torso, with your feet pointing towards the ceiling.

Lowering Phase (Eccentric Movement):

- Exhale as you slowly lower your legs back to the starting position. Control the descent, keeping your legs straight and your core engaged.

- Lower your legs until they are just above the ground, ensuring your lower back remains pressed into the mat. Avoid letting your feet touch the ground to maintain tension in your abdominal muscles.

Repetition:

- Repeat the movement for the desired number of repetitions. Aim for 10-15 repetitions to start, gradually increasing as you build strength and endurance.

Common Mistakes to Avoid:

- **Arching the lower back**: Keep your lower back pressed into the mat to avoid placing undue stress on your spine.

- **Using momentum**: Perform the exercise in a controlled manner, avoiding the use of momentum to lift or lower your legs.

- **Inadequate range of motion**: Lower your legs as close to the ground as possible without letting your lower back lift off the mat.

Tips for Beginners:

- **Bent-knee leg raises**: If straight-leg raises are too challenging, start with bent-knee leg raises. Keep your knees bent at a 90-degree angle and perform the exercise with the same controlled movement.

- **Support with hands**: Place your hands under your glutes or lower back for added support and to help maintain proper form.

- **Shorter range of motion**: Begin with a smaller range of motion, lifting your legs only partway, and gradually increase the range as you build strength.

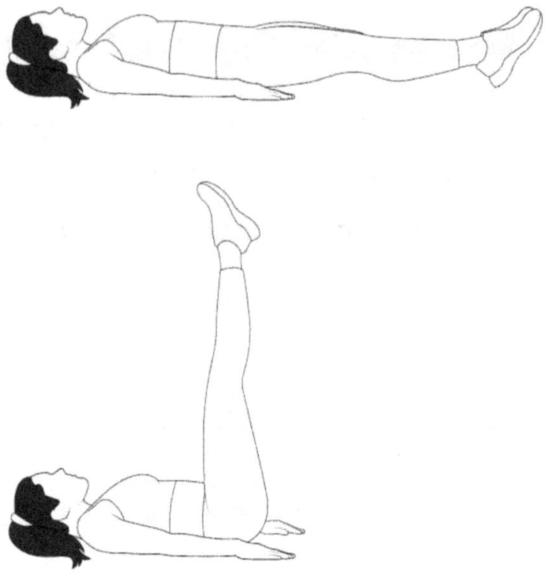

Bicycle Crunches: Engages entire abdominal area.

Starting Position:

Lie flat on your back on an exercise mat with your legs extended and your hands placed lightly behind your head. Engage your core by pulling your belly button towards your spine and lifting your head, shoulders, and feet slightly off the ground.

Execution:

Twisting and Pedaling Movement:

- Inhale deeply as you prepare to begin. Simultaneously bend your right knee and bring it towards your chest while twisting your torso to bring your left elbow towards your right knee. Your left leg should remain extended and hover above the ground.

- Exhale as you twist and contract your obliques, touching your elbow to your knee if possible.

Alternating Sides:

- Inhale as you return to the starting position with your shoulders and feet still off the ground.

- Exhale as you repeat the movement on the opposite side: bend your left knee towards your chest while twisting your torso to bring your right elbow towards your left knee, extending your right leg straight and hovering above the ground.

- Continue to alternate sides in a controlled, bicycle-pedaling motion.

Maintaining Form:

- Keep your core engaged throughout the movement to prevent your lower back from arching off the mat.

- Avoid pulling on your neck with your hands. Your hands should support your head lightly without causing strain.

Common Mistakes to Avoid:

- **Using momentum**: Perform the exercise slowly and deliberately to maximize muscle engagement and avoid relying on momentum.

- **Pulling on the neck**: Keep your hands lightly behind your head and focus on twisting your torso, not pulling your head forward.

- **Inadequate range of motion**: Fully extend each leg and bring each knee towards your chest to ensure a complete range of motion.

Tips for Beginners:

- **Feet on the ground**: Start with your feet on the ground and perform the twisting motion with your upper body only. Gradually progress to lifting your feet off the ground.

- **Shorter duration**: Perform the exercise for a shorter period or fewer repetitions, gradually increasing as you build strength and endurance.

- **Support your lower back**: If you experience discomfort in your lower back, place a small rolled towel under your lower back for support.

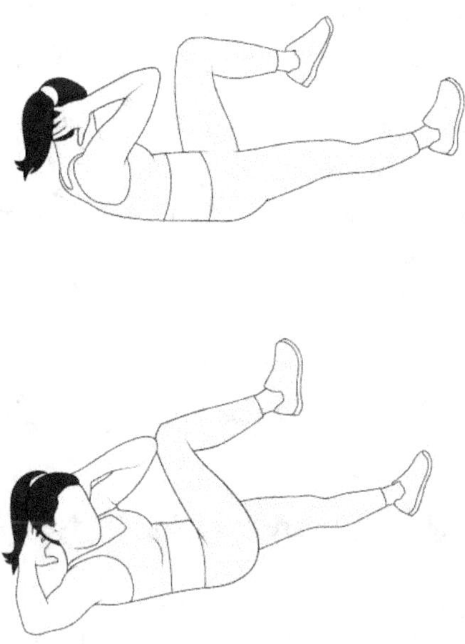

Mountain Climbers: Combines core and cardiovascular benefits.

Starting Position:

Begin in a high plank position with your hands placed shoulder-width apart on the floor, directly under your shoulders. Your body should form a straight line from head to heels. Engage your core to maintain a stable, neutral spine, and keep your shoulders, hips, and ankles aligned.

Execution:

Running Motion:

- Inhale as you prepare to start. Quickly drive your right knee towards your chest while keeping your left leg extended.

- Exhale as you switch legs, driving your left knee towards your chest while extending your right leg back. Continue to alternate legs in a quick, running-like motion.

Maintaining Form:

- Keep your core engaged throughout the exercise to prevent your hips from sagging or lifting too high.

- Ensure your hands remain directly under your shoulders, and your shoulders are over your wrists to maintain proper alignment.

- Move your legs quickly and smoothly, maintaining a steady pace.

Common Mistakes to Avoid:

- **Sagging hips**: Keep your core tight to prevent your hips from dropping, which can strain your lower back.

- **Hips too high**: Maintain a straight line from head to heels, avoiding lifting your hips too high.

- **Improper hand placement**: Keep your hands directly under your shoulders to maintain stability and proper form.

Tips for Beginners:

- **Slower pace**: Start at a slower pace to focus on form and gradually increase your speed as you become more comfortable with the movement.

- **Alternating step**: Instead of a running motion, perform a slower, controlled step by bringing one knee towards your chest at a time.

- **Support your wrists**: If you experience discomfort in your wrists, place your hands on an elevated surface like a bench or step to reduce the pressure.

Advanced Core Work

- Dragon Flags

- Hanging Leg Raises

- Ab Wheel Rollouts

- Side Planks with Leg Lift

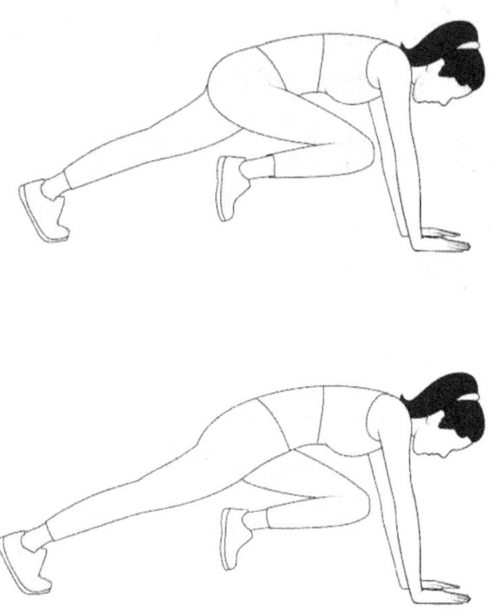

CHAPTER **6**

CARDIO

Effective Bodyweight Cardio Exercises

Burpees: Full-body cardio and strength exercise.

Starting Position:

Stand upright with your feet shoulder-width apart and your arms relaxed at your sides. Engage your core and maintain a straight posture.

Execution:

Squatting Down:

- Inhale as you bend your knees and lower your body into a squat position. Place your hands on the floor directly in front of you, just inside your feet.

Jumping Back (Plank Position):

- Exhale as you jump your feet back to land in a high plank position, with your body forming a straight line from head to heels. Keep your core engaged, and avoid letting your hips sag or rise too high.

Performing a Push-Up:

- Inhale as you lower your chest to the floor by bending your elbows and performing a push-up. Keep your elbows close to your body.

- Exhale as you push through your palms to extend your arms and return to the high plank position.

Jumping Forward:

- Inhale as you jump your feet forward to land just outside your hands, returning to the squat position. Keep your core tight and your back straight.

Jumping Up:

- Exhale as you explosively jump into the air, reaching your arms overhead. Fully extend your body at the top of the jump.

- Land softly with your knees slightly bent to absorb the impact, immediately transitioning into the next repetition.

Maintaining Form:

- Throughout the movement, keep your core engaged to protect your lower back.

- Ensure smooth transitions between each phase of the burpee to maintain a steady rhythm.

Common Mistakes to Avoid:

- **Sagging hips in the plank position**: Keep your core tight to maintain a straight line from head to heels.

- **Incorrect hand placement**: Place your hands directly under your shoulders during the plank and push-up phases.

- **Rushing the movement**: Focus on performing each phase with control and proper form rather than speed.

Tips for Beginners:

- **Modified burpees**: Start with a modified version by stepping your feet back one at a time into the plank position instead of jumping.

- **No push-up**: If the push-up is too challenging, perform the burpee without the push-up phase, focusing on the squat, plank, and jump components.

- **Lower jump**: Perform a smaller jump at the end, gradually increasing the height as you build strength and confidence.

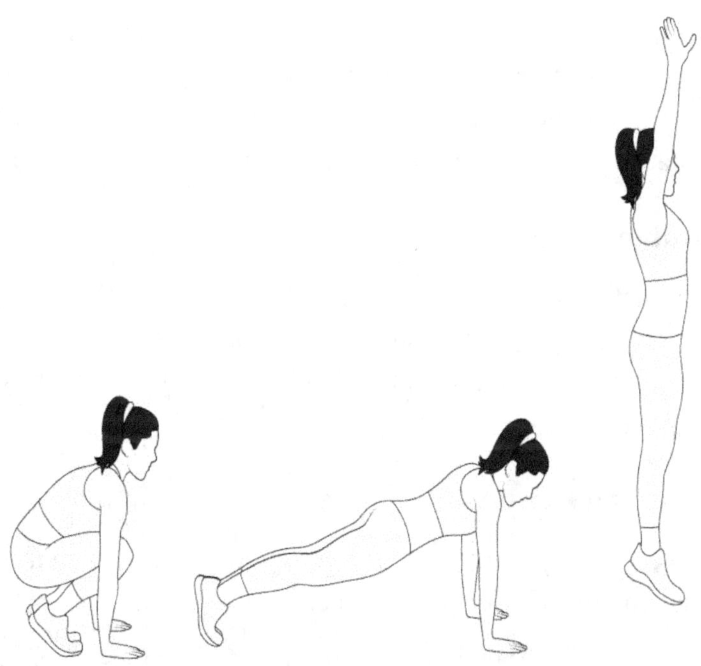

Jumping Jacks: Improves cardiovascular health.

Starting Position:

Stand upright with your feet together and your arms resting at your sides. Engage your core and maintain a straight posture.

Execution:

Jumping Phase:

- Inhale as you prepare to jump. Simultaneously, jump both feet out to the sides, slightly wider than shoulder-width apart, while raising your arms above your head. Your hands should almost touch at the top.

Returning Phase:

- Exhale as you quickly jump your feet back together, bringing your arms back down to your sides. Return to the starting position, maintaining a smooth and controlled movement.

Maintaining Form:

- Keep your core engaged throughout the exercise to maintain stability and balance.

- Ensure your knees are slightly bent as you jump to absorb the impact and reduce stress on your joints.

- Move your arms and legs in a coordinated manner, maintaining a steady rhythm.

Common Mistakes to Avoid:

- **Flailing arms**: Keep your arm movements controlled and coordinated with your leg movements.

- **Straight legs**: Avoid locking your knees. Keep them slightly bent to absorb the impact of each jump.

- **Slouching**: Maintain an upright posture with your chest lifted and shoulders back.

Tips for Beginners:

- **Slower pace**: Start at a slower pace to focus on proper form and gradually increase your speed as you become more comfortable with the movement.

- **Lower intensity**: If jumping is too intense, step one foot out to the side at a time while raising your arms, then return to the starting position.

- **Shorter duration**: Perform jumping jacks for a shorter period, such as 20-30 seconds, and gradually increase the duration as your endurance improves.

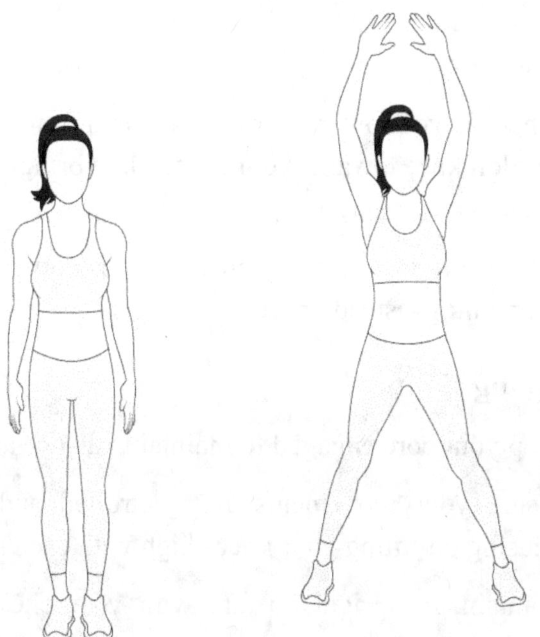

High Knees: Increases heart rate and leg strength.

Starting Position:

Stand upright with your feet hip-width apart. Engage your core and keep your back straight. Your arms should be relaxed at your sides.

Execution:

Lifting Phase:

- Inhale as you prepare to start. Quickly drive your right knee towards your chest, lifting it as high as possible.

- Simultaneously, bring your left arm up to shoulder height, similar to a running motion.

Switching Legs:

- Exhale as you lower your right leg and immediately drive your left knee towards your chest while bringing your right arm up.

- Continue to alternate legs in a quick, running-like motion, maintaining a steady rhythm.

Maintaining Form:

- Keep your core engaged to maintain balance and stability.

- Ensure your movements are controlled and deliberate, focusing on lifting your knees high with each step.

- Maintain an upright posture with your chest lifted and shoulders back.

Common Mistakes to Avoid:

- **Slouching**: Keep your back straight and chest lifted to avoid putting strain on your lower back.

- **Low knee lift**: Aim to lift your knees as high as possible, ideally to hip level, to maximize the effectiveness of the exercise.

- **Using momentum**: Perform the movement with control, ensuring that each knee lift is driven by your muscles rather than momentum.

Tips for Beginners:

- **Slower pace**: Start at a slower pace to focus on proper form and gradually increase your speed as you become more comfortable with the movement.

- **Lower knee lift**: If lifting your knees to hip height is too challenging, start with a lower knee lift and gradually increase the height as your strength and endurance improve.

- **Shorter duration**: Perform high knees for a shorter period, such as 20-30 seconds, and gradually increase the duration as your fitness level improves.

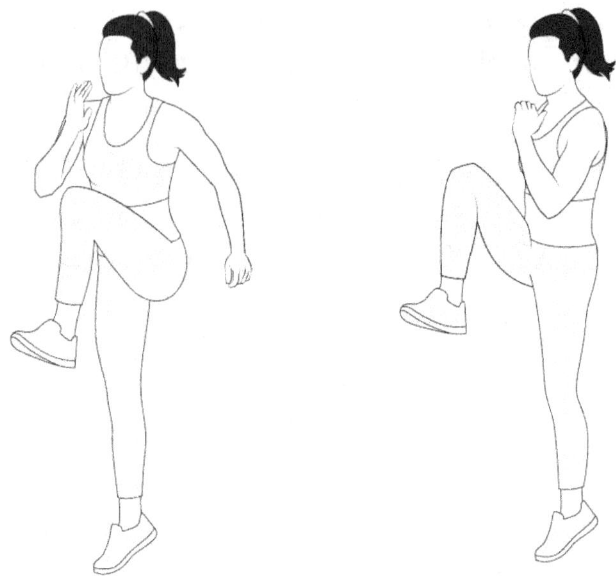

Tuck jumps: Improves cardiovascular health.

Starting Position:

Stand upright with your feet shoulder-width apart and your knees slightly bent. Engage your core and keep your chest lifted. Your arms should be relaxed at your sides.

Execution:

Jumping Phase:

- Inhale as you prepare to jump. Bend your knees slightly to get into a quarter squat position.

- Exhale as you explosively jump straight up into the air. Drive your knees towards your chest, aiming to tuck them as high as possible.

Tucking Phase:

- At the peak of your jump, bring your knees up towards your chest, wrapping your arms around your knees briefly if needed.

- Keep your core engaged to help lift your knees and maintain balance.

Landing Phase:

- Land softly on the balls of your feet, immediately bending your knees to absorb the impact. This helps to protect your joints and prepare you for the next jump.

- Ensure your feet return to shoulder-width apart and your body is ready to jump again if performing multiple repetitions.

Maintaining Form:

- Keep your core tight throughout the exercise to stabilize your body and maintain control.

- Focus on landing softly and quietly to reduce the impact on your joints.

- Maintain an upright posture with your chest lifted and shoulders back.

Common Mistakes to Avoid:

- Flat-footed landing: Always land on the balls of your feet and bend your knees to absorb the impact.

- Leaning forward or backward: Maintain an upright posture to avoid straining your lower back.

- Incomplete knee tuck: Aim to bring your knees as high as possible towards your chest for maximum effectiveness.

Tips for Beginners:

- Lower jump height: If tuck jumps are too challenging, start with a lower jump height and gradually increase as you build strength and confidence.

- Practice squats: Build strength and proper form by practicing squats and squat jumps before progressing to tuck jumps.

- Shorter duration: Perform fewer repetitions or shorter sets, gradually increasing the number as your fitness improves.

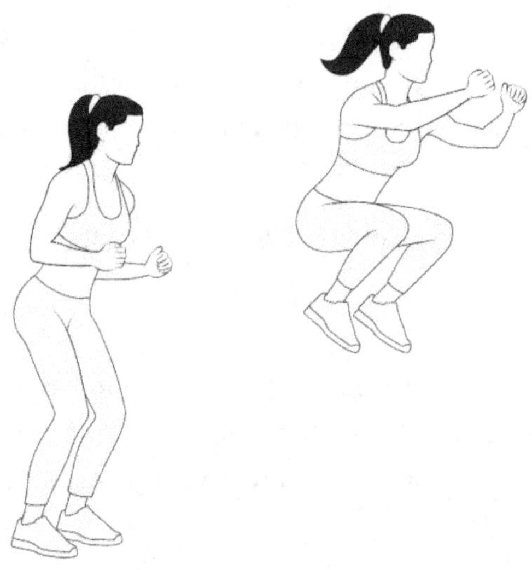

Jump Squats: Boosts explosive power and cardio fitness.

Starting Position:

Stand upright with your feet shoulder-width apart and your arms relaxed at your sides. Engage your core and keep your chest lifted and shoulders back.

Execution:

Squatting Phase:

- Inhale as you lower your body into a squat position by bending your knees and pushing your hips back. Your thighs should be parallel to the ground, and your knees should be directly above your toes.

- Keep your back straight and your core engaged to maintain proper alignment.

Jumping Phase:

- Exhale as you explode upward from the squat position, pushing through your heels and extending your legs. Use the power from your legs and core to propel yourself into the air.

- Swing your arms overhead to help generate momentum.

Landing Phase:

- Land softly on the balls of your feet, immediately bending your knees to absorb the impact and return to the squat position. This helps to protect your joints and prepare you for the next jump.

- Ensure your feet return to shoulder-width apart and your body is ready to jump again if performing multiple repetitions.

Maintaining Form:

- Keep your core tight throughout the exercise to stabilize your body and maintain control.

- Focus on landing softly and quietly to reduce the impact on your joints.

- Maintain an upright posture with your chest lifted and shoulders back.

Common Mistakes to Avoid:

- **Flat-footed landing**: Always land on the balls of your feet and bend your knees to absorb the impact.

- **Leaning forward**: Keep your chest up and back straight to avoid straining your lower back.

- **Inadequate depth**: Lower your body into a full squat position to maximize the effectiveness of the exercise.

Tips for Beginners:

- **Lower jump height**: If jump squats are too challenging, start with a lower jump height and gradually increase as you build strength and confidence.

- **Practice squats**: Build strength and proper form by practicing regular squats before progressing to jump squats.

- **Shorter duration**: Perform fewer repetitions or shorter sets, gradually increasing the number as your fitness improves.

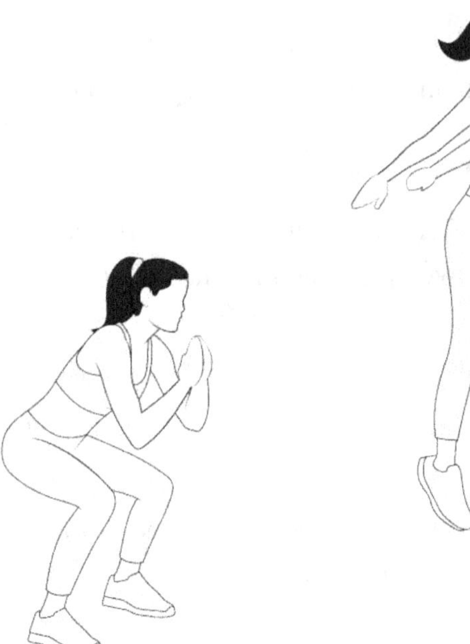

CHAPTER 7

FLEXIBILITY/STRETCHING EXERCISES

Importance of Flexibility

- Reduces the risk of injuries.

- Improves posture and balance.

- Enhances overall movement efficiency.

Key Stretching Exercises

Hamstring Stretch*:* Improves flexibility in the back of the legs.

Starting Position:

Begin by standing upright with your feet hip-width apart. Ensure you have enough space around you to perform the stretch without any obstructions.

Execution:

Standing Hamstring Stretch:

- **Inhale and Prepare**: Stand tall, engaging your core to maintain balance. Keep your back straight and shoulders relaxed.

- **Extend Your Right Leg**: Step your right foot slightly forward, resting your heel on the ground with your toes pointing upwards. Your left knee should be slightly bent for stability.

- **Hinge at the Hips**: Exhale as you hinge at your hips, keeping your back straight.

Lower your upper body towards your extended right leg. Reach your hands towards your right foot. You should feel a stretch along the back of your right thigh.

- **Hold the Stretch**: Hold this position for 20-30 seconds, breathing deeply and steadily. Ensure that you do not round your back; keep it straight to avoid straining your lower back.

- **Switch Sides**: Inhale as you slowly return to the starting position. Repeat the stretch on your left leg, stepping your left foot forward and hinging at the hips to reach towards your left foot.

Seated Hamstring Stretch:

- **Inhale and Prepare**: Sit on the floor with your legs extended straight in front of you. Engage your core and sit up tall, ensuring your back is straight.

- **Extend Your Arms**: Reach your arms forward towards your toes. If you can't reach your toes, reach towards your shins or ankles.

- **Hinge at the Hips**: Exhale as you hinge at your hips, lowering your upper body towards your legs. Focus on maintaining a straight back.

- **Hold the Stretch**: Hold this position for 20-30 seconds, breathing deeply and steadily. You should feel a stretch along the back of your thighs.

Common Mistakes to Avoid:

- **Rounding the back**: Keep your back straight to avoid straining your lower back and to ensure an effective stretch.

- **Bouncing**: Avoid bouncing into the stretch, as this can cause muscle strain. Use slow, controlled movements.

- **Overstretching**: Do not push your body beyond its comfort zone. Stretch until you feel mild tension, not pain.

Tips for Beginners:

- **Use a towel or strap**: If you have difficulty reaching your toes, use a towel or yoga strap around your feet to assist in the stretch.

- **Gentle stretch**: Start with a gentle stretch and gradually increase the depth as your flexibility improves.

- **Regular practice**: Incorporate hamstring stretches into your routine regularly to improve flexibility over time.

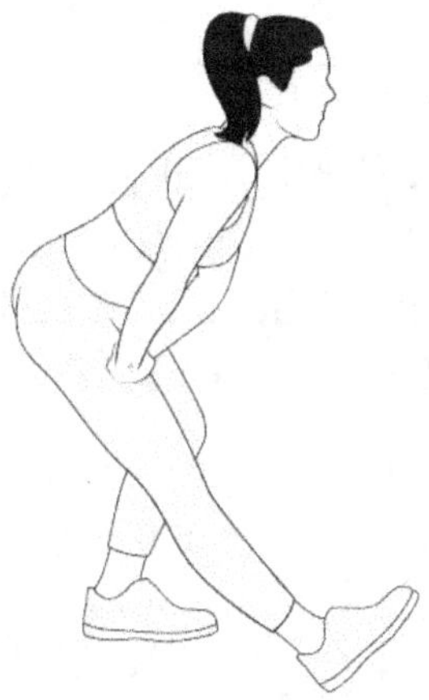

Quadriceps Stretch: Targets the front of the thighs.

Starting Position:

Begin by standing upright with your feet hip-width apart. Ensure you have enough space around you to perform the stretch without any obstructions. You may use a wall or chair for balance if needed.

Execution:

Standing Quadriceps Stretch:

- **Inhale and Prepare**: Stand tall, engaging your core to maintain balance. Keep your back straight and shoulders relaxed.

- **Lift Your Right Foot**: Bend your right knee and lift your right foot towards your glutes. Reach back with your right hand to grasp your right ankle. Use your left hand to hold onto a wall or chair for balance if necessary.

- **Hold Your Ankle**: Gently pull your right ankle towards your glutes, feeling a stretch along the front of your thigh. Ensure that your knees are close together and not flaring out to the side.

- **Maintain Proper Alignment**: Keep your hips square and push them slightly forward to deepen the stretch. Avoid arching your back; maintain a neutral spine.

- **Hold the Stretch**: Hold this position for 20-30 seconds, breathing deeply and steadily. Ensure that you do not bounce; keep the stretch steady and controlled.

- **Switch Sides**: Slowly release your right ankle and return to the starting position. Repeat the stretch on your left leg, lifting your left foot towards your glutes and grasping your left ankle with your left hand.

Lying Quadriceps Stretch (alternative):

- **Lie on Your Side**: Lie on your left side with your legs stacked and straight. Support your head with your left arm.

- **Lift Your Right Foot**: Bend your right knee and bring your right foot towards your glutes. Reach back with your right hand to grasp your right ankle.

- **Hold Your Ankle**: Gently pull your right ankle towards your glutes, feeling a stretch along the front of your thigh. Keep your knees close together.

- **Maintain Proper Alignment**: Keep your hips aligned and avoid arching your back.

- **Hold the Stretch**: Hold this position for 20-30 seconds, breathing deeply and steadily.

- **Switch Sides**: Roll onto your right side and repeat the stretch with your left leg.

Common Mistakes to Avoid:

- **Arching the back**: Keep your spine neutral to avoid straining your lower back.

- **Knees flaring out**: Ensure your knees remain close together to maximize the effectiveness of the stretch.

- **Bouncing**: Avoid bouncing into the stretch, as this can cause muscle strain. Use slow, controlled movements.

Tips for Beginners:

- **Use a strap**: If you have difficulty reaching your ankle, use a yoga strap or towel around your ankle to assist in the stretch.

- **Gentle stretch**: Start with a gentle stretch and gradually increase the depth as your flexibility improves.

- **Regular practice**: Incorporate quadriceps stretches into your routine regularly to improve flexibility over time.

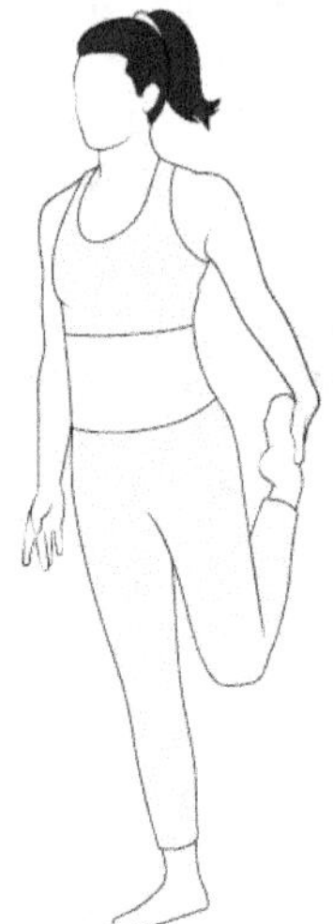 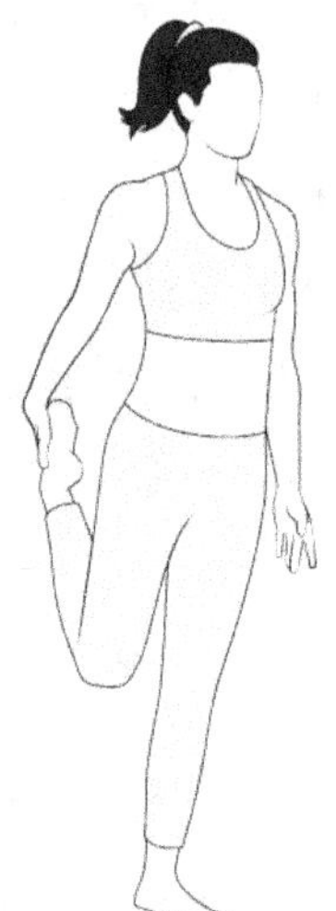

Chest Opener: Enhances flexibility in the chest and shoulders.

Starting Position:

Stand upright with your feet hip-width apart. Ensure you have enough space around you to perform the stretch without any obstructions. You can also perform this stretch while seated if preferred.

Execution:

Standing Chest Opener:

- **Inhale and Prepare**: Stand tall, engaging your core to maintain balance. Keep your back straight and shoulders relaxed.

- **Interlace Your Fingers**: Reach behind your back and interlace your fingers. If this is challenging, you can hold a towel or yoga strap between your hands to assist with the stretch.

- **Lift Your Arms**: Exhale as you gently lift your interlaced hands away from your back. Keep your arms straight, but avoid locking your elbows.

- **Open Your Chest**: Push your chest forward and squeeze your shoulder blades together, feeling a stretch across your chest and the front of your shoulders.

Keep your neck neutral, and avoid tilting your head forward or backward.

- **Hold the Stretch:** Hold this position for 20-30 seconds, breathing deeply and steadily. Ensure the stretch is felt in your chest without causing pain or discomfort.

- **Release and Relax:** Slowly lower your arms back to the starting position and release your hands.

Alternative Version:

Doorway Chest Opener:

- **Find a Doorway**: Stand in a doorway with your feet hip-width apart.

- **Position Your Arms**: Place your forearms on each side of the doorway, elbows at shoulder height.

- **Step Forward**: Gently step forward with one foot, feeling a stretch across your chest as your body moves forward.

- **Hold and Switch**: Hold the stretch for 20-30 seconds, then switch feet and repeat.

Common Mistakes to Avoid:

- **Arching the back**: Keep your spine neutral to avoid straining your lower back.

- **Locking elbows**: Keep your arms straight, but avoid locking your elbows to prevent joint strain.

- **Tilting the head**: Maintain a neutral neck position to avoid straining your neck.

Tips for Beginners:

- **Use a towel or strap**: If you have difficulty interlacing your fingers behind your back, use a towel or yoga strap to assist in the stretch.

- **Gentle stretch**: Start with a gentle stretch and gradually increase the intensity as your flexibility improves.

- **Regular practice**: Incorporate chest opener stretches into your routine regularly to improve flexibility and counteract the effects of poor posture

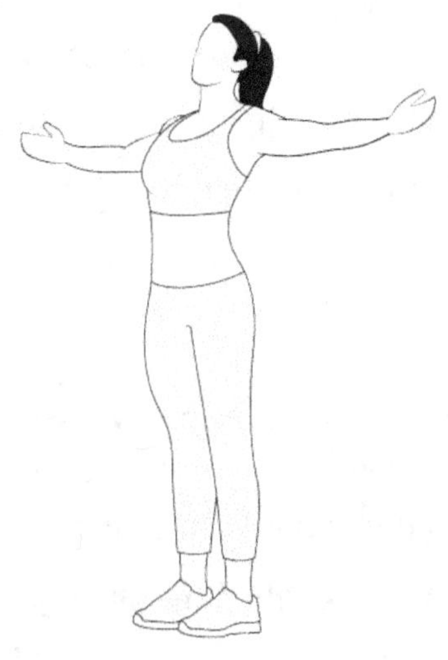

Cat-Cow Stretch: Increases spinal flexibility.

Starting Position:

Begin on all fours in a tabletop position. Ensure your wrists are directly under your shoulders and your knees are directly under your hips. Spread your fingers wide for stability and engage your core.

Execution:

Cow Pose (Inhale):

- **Inhale Deeply:** As you inhale, drop your belly towards the mat. Lift your chin and chest, and gaze up toward the ceiling. Allow your shoulder blades to spread apart.

- **Tilt Your Pelvis:** Tilt your pelvis back, lifting your tailbone towards the ceiling to create a gentle arch in your back.

Cat Pose (Exhale):

- **Exhale Fully:** As you exhale, draw your belly to your spine and round your back towards the ceiling. Tuck your chin to your chest, and let your head drop.

- **Tuck Your Pelvis:** Tilt your pelvis forward, curling your tailbone under to enhance the stretch along your spine.

Flowing Movement:

- **Smooth Transition:** Continue to flow smoothly between Cow Pose and Cat Pose, matching your breath to your movements. Inhale as you move into Cow Pose and exhale as you transition into Cat Pose.

- **Repeat the Sequence:** Perform the stretch for 5-10 breath cycles, or as long as it feels comfortable, allowing each movement to flow naturally into the next.

Maintaining Form:

- **Engage Your Core:** Keep your core engaged throughout the movement to support your spine.

- **Move Slowly:** Perform the movements slowly and with control, focusing on the full range of motion.

- **Align Your Joints:** Ensure your wrists remain directly under your shoulders and your knees under your hips throughout the exercise.

Common Mistakes to Avoid:

- **Rapid Movements:** Avoid performing the movements too quickly; instead, focus on slow, controlled transitions to maximize the stretch.

- **Excessive Arching:** Do not over-arch your back in Cow Pose or over-round it in Cat Pose. Aim for a gentle, comfortable range of motion.

- **Poor Alignment:** Keep your hands and knees properly aligned to prevent strain on your joints.

Tips for Beginners:

- **Comfortable Surface:** Perform the stretch on a yoga mat or soft surface to protect your knees and wrists.

- **Focus on Breath:** Use your breath to guide the movements, enhancing the mind-body connection.

- **Regular Practice:** Incorporate Cat-Cow stretches into your daily routine to improve spinal flexibility and relieve tension.

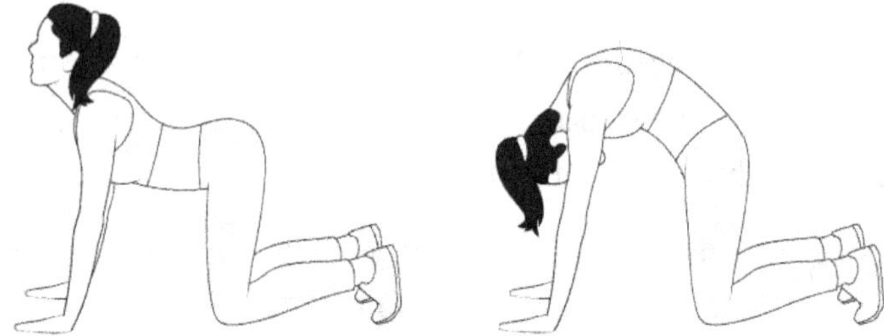

CHAPTER **8**

A SAMPLE AND EXPLANATION OF A CIRCUIT

Understanding Circuit Training

Circuit training is a highly efficient workout method that combines multiple exercises performed in a specific sequence with minimal rest between each exercise. This training approach enhances cardiovascular fitness, muscular endurance, and overall workout efficiency, making it an excellent choice for those looking to maximize their fitness results in a limited amount of time.

Combines Multiple Exercises:

In a typical circuit training session, you'll perform a variety of exercises that target different muscle groups. This could include a mix of strength training moves, such as push-ups, squats, and lunges, along with cardiovascular exercises like jumping jacks, burpees, and mountain climbers. Each exercise is performed for a set period (e.g., 30 seconds) or a specific number of repetitions before moving on to the next exercise.

Performed in Sequence with Minimal Rest:

The exercises in a circuit are performed back-to-back with minimal rest in between, usually no more than 15-30 seconds. This continuous movement keeps your heart rate elevated throughout the workout, which enhances cardiovascular conditioning and burns more calories. The brief rest periods also challenge your muscular endurance, as your muscles have less time to recover between exercises.

Enhances Cardiovascular Fitness:

The combination of strength and cardio exercises in circuit training significantly boosts cardiovascular fitness. By continuously moving from one exercise to the next, your heart and lungs work harder to supply oxygen to your muscles. This improves your overall cardiovascular health, increases your aerobic capacity, and enhances your endurance.

Improves Muscular Endurance:

Muscular endurance is the ability of your muscles to perform repetitive contractions over an extended period. Circuit training improves muscular endurance by incorporating a variety of strength exercises with minimal rest. This challenges your muscles to sustain effort for longer periods, leading to increased stamina and resistance to fatigue.

Overall Workout Efficiency:

Circuit training is highly efficient because it combines both strength and cardio elements in a single workout. This makes it ideal for those with limited time, as you can achieve a comprehensive full-body workout in as little as 20-30 minutes. Additionally, the variety of exercises prevents boredom and keeps your body guessing, which can help to avoid plateaus and continue making progress.

Sample Circuit

1. **Push-Ups**: 30 seconds
2. **Squats**: 30 seconds
3. **Plank**: 30 seconds
4. **Burpees**: 30 seconds
5. **Mountain Climbers**: 30 seconds
6. **Rest**: 1 minute

Repeat for 3-5 rounds.

30-DAY DETAILED WORKOUT PLAN

Instructions:

- Perform each exercise with proper form.

- Adjust the intensity as needed.

- Ensure proper warm-up before each workout and cool down afterward.

Week 1

Day 1: Full Body Introduction

1. Jumping Jacks - 30 seconds
2. Squats - 15 reps
3. Push-Ups - 10 reps (use knee modification if needed)
4. Cat-Cow Stretch - 10 cycles
5. Plank - 20 seconds

Day 2: Lower Body Focus

1. Jump Squats - 10 reps
2. Lunges - 10 reps per leg
3. Calf Raises - 15 reps
4. Hamstring Stretch - 30 seconds per leg
5. Quadriceps Stretch - 30 seconds per leg

Day 3: Upper Body and Core

1. Pike Push-Ups - 10 reps
2. Mountain Climbers - 30 seconds
3. Leg Raises - 10 reps
4. Russian Twists - 15 reps per side
5. Chest Opener Stretch - 30 seconds

Day 4: Rest Day

Day 5: Cardio and Core

1. High Knees - 30 seconds
2. Bicycle Crunches - 15 reps per side
3. Burpees - 10 reps
4. Plank - 30 seconds
5. Cat-Cow Stretch - 10 cycles

Day 6: Full Body

1. Jumping Jacks - 30 seconds
2. Step-Ups - 10 reps per leg
3. Push-Ups - 10 reps
4. Tuck Jumps - 10 reps
5. Hip Flexor Stretch - 30 seconds per side

Day 7: Rest Day

Week 2

Day 8: Lower Body Strength

1. Squats - 15 reps
2. Lunges - 12 reps per leg
3. Calf Raises - 15 reps
4. Hamstring Stretch - 30 seconds per leg
5. Quadriceps Stretch - 30 seconds per leg

Day 9: Core and Cardio

1. High Knees - 30 seconds
2. Bicycle Crunches - 20 reps per side
3. Plank - 40 seconds
4. Mountain Climbers - 30 seconds
5. Cat-Cow Stretch - 10 cycles

Day 10: Upper Body

1. Pike Push-Ups - 12 reps
2. Push-Ups - 12 reps
3. Chest Opener Stretch - 30 seconds
4. Russian Twists - 20 reps per side
5. Leg Raises - 15 reps

Day 11: Rest Day

Day 12: Full Body Conditioning

1. Jumping Jacks - 40 seconds
2. Jump Squats - 12 reps
3. Step-Ups - 12 reps per leg
4. Burpees - 12 reps

5. Hip Flexor Stretch - 30 seconds per side

Day 13: Lower Body and Core

1. Squats - 15 reps
2. Lunges - 12 reps per leg
3. Plank - 45 seconds
4. Bicycle Crunches - 20 reps per side
5. Hamstring Stretch - 30 seconds per leg

Day 14: Rest Day

Week 3

Day 15: Upper Body Strength

1. Pike Push-Ups - 15 reps
2. Push-Ups - 15 reps
3. Chest Opener Stretch - 30 seconds
4. Russian Twists - 20 reps per side
5. Leg Raises - 15 reps

Day 16: Cardio Blast

1. High Knees - 40 seconds
2. Mountain Climbers - 40 seconds
3. Tuck Jumps - 15 reps
4. Jumping Jacks - 40 seconds
5. Cat-Cow Stretch - 10 cycles

Day 17: Lower Body Focus

1. Squats - 20 reps
2. Step-Ups - 15 reps per leg
3. Calf Raises - 20 reps
4. Quadriceps Stretch - 30 seconds per leg

5. Hamstring Stretch - 30 seconds per leg

Day 18: Rest Day

Day 19: Core and Stability

1. Plank - 50 seconds
2. Bicycle Crunches - 25 reps per side
3. Russian Twists - 25 reps per side
4. Leg Raises - 20 reps
5. Hip Flexor Stretch - 30 seconds per side

Day 20: Full Body Workout

1. Jumping Jacks - 45 seconds
2. Burpees - 15 reps
3. Lunges - 15 reps per leg
4. Push-Ups - 15 reps
5. Cat-Cow Stretch - 10 cycles

Day 21: Rest Day

Week 4

Day 22: Lower Body Power

1. Squats - 20 reps
2. Jump Squats - 15 reps
3. Step-Ups - 15 reps per leg
4. Calf Raises - 20 reps
5. Hamstring Stretch - 30 seconds per leg

Day 23: Cardio and Core

1. High Knees - 45 seconds
2. Mountain Climbers - 45 seconds

3. Bicycle Crunches - 25 reps per side
4. Plank - 60 seconds
5. Hip Flexor Stretch - 30 seconds per side

Day 24: Upper Body Strength

1. Pike Push-Ups - 15 reps
2. Push-Ups - 15 reps
3. Chest Opener Stretch - 30 seconds
4. Russian Twists - 25 reps per side
5. Leg Raises - 20 reps

Day 25: Rest Day

Day 26: Full Body Blast

1. Jumping Jacks - 50 seconds
2. Burpees - 15 reps
3. Tuck Jumps - 15 reps
4. Squats - 20 reps
5. Cat-Cow Stretch - 10 cycles

Day 27: Lower Body and Core

1. Lunges - 20 reps per leg
2. Step-Ups - 20 reps per leg
3. Plank - 60 seconds
4. Bicycle Crunches - 25 reps per side
5. Hamstring Stretch - 30 seconds per leg

Day 28: Rest Day

Day 29: Upper Body and Cardio

1. High Knees - 50 seconds
2. Pike Push-Ups - 20 reps

3. Push-Ups - 20 reps
4. Mountain Climbers - 50 seconds
5. Chest Opener Stretch - 30 seconds

Day 30: Final Full Body Workout

1. Jumping Jacks - 60 seconds
2. Squats - 25 reps
3. Burpees - 20 reps
4. Russian Twists - 30 reps per side
5. Cat-Cow Stretch - 10 cycles

CONCLUSION

Bodyweight training offers a sustainable, versatile, and effective way to achieve your fitness goals. By incorporating the exercises and routines outlined in this book, you can build strength, improve cardiovascular health, enhance flexibility, and develop a well-rounded fitness regimen that fits seamlessly into your lifestyle. Remember, consistency is key. Stay dedicated, listen to your body, and enjoy the journey to a healthier, fitter you.

If you found this book helpful, I'd be very appreciative if you left a favorable review for the book on Amazon!

RESOURCES

10 benefits of bodyweight exercises, according to experts. (n.d.). Nike.com. https://www.nike.com/a/bodyweight-exercise-benefits

10 HIIT workouts for beginners that will burn calories and boost your metabolism. (2023, August 15). TODAY.com.

https://www.today.com/health/diet-fitness/hiit-workouts-for-beginners-rcna99970

Yeung, A. J. (2023, May 6). 7 bodyweight exercise mistakes to avoid after 40. *Eat This Not That.* htCPT, J. M. (2019, January 3). How to set fitness goals you'll actually achieve, according to top trainers. *SELF.*

https://www.self.com/story/how-to-set-realistic-fitness-goalstps://www.eatthis.com/bodyweight-e xercise-mistakes-to-avoid-after-40/

Exercises to improve your core strength. (2023, August 25). Mayo Clinic. https://www.mayoclinic.org/healthy-lifestyle/fitness/in-depth/core-strength/art-20546851

CPT, A. M. W., CPT, J. M., & CPT, C. S. (2023, January 4). 31 leg exercises at home that require no equipment. *SELF.*

https://www.self.com/gallery/killer-legs-no-gear-required-slideshow

Squat progression. (n.d.). http://www.startbodyweight.com/p/squat-progression.html

Set, S. F. (2024, May 7). *The ultimate upper body bodyweight workout.* SET FOR SET.

https://www.setforset.com/blogs/news/upper-body-bodyweight-workout

Bathurst, J., & Bathurst, J. (2024, January 26). *The Push-up progression Plan (Get your first push-up!).* Nerd Fitness. https://www.nerdfitness.com/blog/push-up-progression-plan/

Cpt, T. R. B. (2021, April 23). *The 8 best agility exercises you can do at home.* Healthline. https://www.healthline.com/health/fitness/agility-exercises

Tweed, K. (2022, August 28). *Yoga Fusion.* WebMD.

https://www.webmd.com/fitness-exercise/a-z/yoga-fusion-classes

Millard, E. (2023, March 9). *The Beginner's Guide to Tabata Workouts.* BODi. https://www.beachbodyondemand.com/blog/tabata-workouts-for-beginners

Animal Flow. (2024, May 15). *Home - Animal flow.* https://animalflow.com/

Mmohabir. (2019, January 8). *10 nutrition rules to follow if you want to build muscle.* Muscle &

Fitness. https://www.muscleandfitness.com/nutrition/gain-mass/10-nutrition-rules-follow-if-you-want-bui ld-muscle/

Dupere, K. (2021, November 2). This guy shared the secrets to his remarkable 8-Year calisthenics transformation. *Men's Health.*

https://www.menshealth.com/fitness/a33941458/calisthenics -exercises-weight-loss-transformatio n-8-year-time-lapse-video/

Robinson, L. (2024, February 5). *How to start exercising and stick to it.* HelpGuide.org. https://www.helpguide.org/articles/healthy-living/how-to-start-exercising-and-stick-to-it.htm

Circuit Training Workouts | Chuze Fitness – Urdailyshop. https://urdailyshop.com/circuit-training-workouts-chuze-fitness/

A Beginner's Guide to High-Intensity Interval Training (HIIT) - chamceul.ind.ws. https://chamceul.ind.ws/2023/04/13/a-beginners-guide-to-high-intensity-interval-training-hiit/

Ultimate Guide: How to Lose Weight in 7 Days Safely and Effectively. https://www.howtolose.online/how-to-lose-weight-in-7-days/

Shouldn't I attempt Russian fighter pull-ups as a beginner? In 2024.

https://myexerciseroutines.com/2023/08/16/shouldnt-i-attempt-russian-fighter-pull-ups-as-a-begi nner/

10 Best Russian Twist Alternatives For A Solid Core [By PT]. https://stronghomegym.com/russian-twist-alternative/

Muscular Endurance - FitnessLife Magazine.

https://fitnesslifemagazine.com/muscular-endurance/